How to get fit

with Reiki and Music

by Francesca Hepton

in collaboration with

Jade Fraser-Boynton

Babili Books

ISBN: 978-1-9999126-2-8

Release your inner champion

霊

+

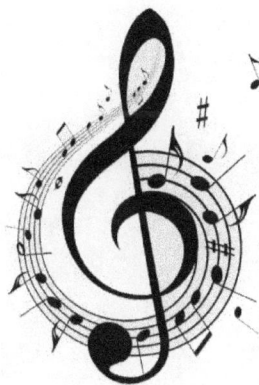

Also by Francesca Hepton
*in the **How to...** series:*

Be Happy
How to Look Young
Save Money
Give up Drinking
Stop Smoking

First published in 2018
by Babili Books

CONTENTS

CONTAINS

FREE GUIDES:

Daily Energy Exercises

Reiki Self-healing Treatment

PLUS
Inspirational playlists

Preface

Most of us are ready to believe in miracles. Most of us feel elated when the hero of a story succeeds against all odds. Most of us... never believe we can beat the odds or experience miracles in our own life.

Why not? Because we stop ourselves through fear and self-doubt before we even start. It's kind of a protection mechanism. You tell yourself that if you stay in your comfort zone nothing bad can happen...

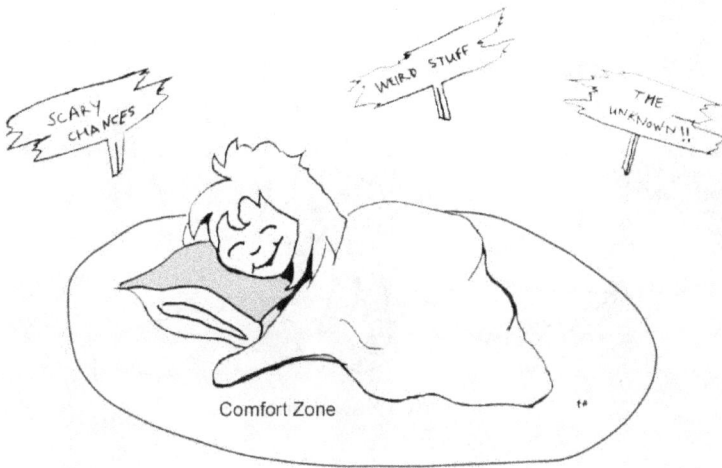

Comfort Zone

Well, something bad does in fact happen and deep down you know it. You become stagnated, fixed in your ways, you stop learning, stop evolving, miss out on all kinds of experiences in life. By not pushing your boundaries you will not create your own miracles or be the hero who succeeds despite the odds being stacked against them. But what if you were given an easy and fulfilling way to achieve your goals (not just in fitness), then your stubborn ego who wants to stay in the comfort zone might be open to listening.

Keeping an open mind is essential to maximising the full power Reiki can offer you in your fitness regime. By embracing its simple practices you can create an environment in your life to facilitate your training and/or healing process.

Let me dig you out of your comfort zone and the hole of self-doubt you are entrenched in. Let me give you wings - or at least open doors in both your mind and life. By being willing to learn a new technique (like the combo of Reiki and music), you are already carving a hole from within your comfort zone to the outside world of possibilities.

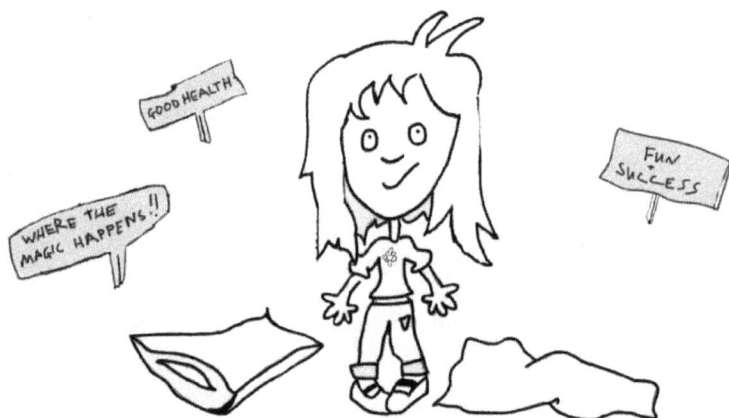

Brave New World

You are probably familiar with music as a motivator thanks to the uplifting and ethereal soundtracks to movies like Rocky, Chariots of Fire and Flashdance. You may be less familiar with Reiki as a motivator and performance enhancer. As with all best practices, I believe it is most beneficial to approach any challenge with an holistic approach. By this I mean an approach that encompasses all factors not just the obvious ones. When we apply this holistic approach to getting fit, I believe we should deal with not just getting the muscular, digestive and respiratory system of the body in shape but also its nervous system, lymphatic system and spiritual system. Reiki (the art of channelling and balancing energy) and music (of all kinds of genres) will be the "complementary" therapies and drivers behind your existing fitness regime or physiotherapy schedule.

Please note that this guide does not provide diets or workouts, you can visit numerous sites, such as LES MILLS which I believe is worth recommending. This guide will however, help you in defining your goals and drawing up your fitness/training plans. It will also help you **find** your motivation and **maintain** your motivation.

If you want to be able to heal from the harmful effects of an accident, win the next marathon, get rid of your bad habits and become a healthy person, lose weight and keep it off, be the most toned or muscular member in your gym or simply get fit to feel great, you can help yourself achieve this with a balanced and energised approach. Does that sound like a million miles away to you right now? Don't worry, the key this book gives you will open the door to achievement one day at a time.

Reiki and music are the facilitators that will help you on this journey. (If you are unfamiliar with Reiki there is an introductory explanation in the first chapter). Reiki will take up just 15 minutes of your day max! And listening to music… well that sounds easy!

Plus I am going to tell you what you need to do to achieve and maintain your state of motivation at the start of the book (so many authors drag you through endless pages before divulging their core message or secret) and then I will provide you with information of how this is all possible will substantive research.

Here's how:

1) All you need to do is 12 to 15 minutes a day of the Reiki energy exercises. I would also recommend you carry out the self-healing treatments to begin with, likewise just 15 minutes, (or visit a reputable Reiki practitioner) until you come through the other side of your

"healing crisis" (it's more of a healing period than a "crisis"). Then just add these to your daily routine as and when you feel the need – when you feel out of balance, or as the usual saying goes, when you feel "out of sorts".

2) Add music to your day, both in and out of the gym or on and off the track. Keep yourself happy, keep yourself motivated. Design your own playlist to suit your training and exercises (remember to keep it slow for the warm ups and cool downs).

3) When you need an extra "boost" to hold plank a little longer or shoot around the last lap, draw on the energy around you through visualisation and intent, as you will learn to do in your daily Reiki energy exercises. You will feel yourself flying and the exercise becomes effortless as you merge with the universal life force around you and its energy pumps through your body.

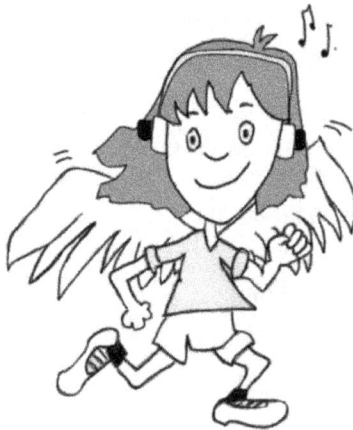

Take flight with Reiki and music

Interested on learning how? Read on and release the power within you through the symbiosis of Reiki and music!

1 – Reiki

Your aim: to get fit

A new approach to getting motivated and staying motivated

Your aim is clear, you want to get fit. Whether it is in terms of gaining muscle mass, improving track times, weight loss, recovering from an injury or as part of your self-improvement overhaul to becoming healthy. With the meditative art of energy channelling (Reiki) and motivational powers of music, this fantastically uplifting and liberating new approach to fitness will help you achieve your targets.

To kick off with, below is a brief insight into the essence of Reiki for those of you who are unfamiliar with the technique, followed by a modern interpretation for those of you who are familiar with traditional Reiki. This modern interpretation helps us to apply Reiki's benefits to our busy schedules and assist us in our endeavours to get fit and healthy.

The traditional face of Reiki

If you ask an average Western man or woman what Reiki means to them, this may conjure up images of farcical gypsy-style women promising to cure you of all ailments by waving their hands around smoky incense-filled rooms to the sounds of jangling bracelets and pan pipes and a little pretend magic. It's no surprise then that this meditative healing practice is shrouded in negative reviews given the charlatans out there practising it. Whatever your preconceptions of Reiki are, wipe the slate clean and approach this subject with fresh eyes. We are taking Reiki back to its pure roots here. Roots based on thousands of years of contemplative wisdom as embodied by the gracious practices of Taoism, Shintoism and Buddhism. Reiki offers a path to mental and physical healing. It is a source of great power and energy, it can be your way to fitness, sustained health and achieving your goals with ease.

Its founder, Mikao Usui, designed Reiki as a form of self-healing (1920s Japan). With Reiki, you draw on an unlimited source of energy that is all around you and circulate it through your body.

(I would like to confirm that although Reiki is associated with spiritual healing and was inspired in part by Tendai Buddhism, Shintoism and Taoism, it is not related to any religion.

REIKI IS NOT A RELIGIOUS PRACTICE! It is a meditative technique.)

What does the word "Reiki" actually mean? Roughly translated from Japanese:

Rei = universal life

Ki = the energy that animates all living things

(pronounced, *ray-key*)

Reiki = energy that flows through all living things / universal life force

Many of us in the Western world are aware of Oriental cultures founded on this technique of drawing on the energy around us... how do you think the masterful Bruce Lee was able to achieve those super cool moves?!

The different names for energy

This "energy" runs through you and surrounds you. The Chinese call it **qi** and channel it through their meridians. **Qi** in Chinese translates as "air" and figuratively as "material **energy**", "life force", or "**energy** flow". **Qi** is the central underlying principle in Chinese traditional medicine and in Chinese martial arts[1] - this forms the basis of acupuncture and shiatsu.

If martial arts or complementary therapy is not your scene perhaps you can affiliate better with the idea of Feng Shui. The art of placement and positioning items around your living environment in such a way that allows the "energy" which is all around us to flow freely and evenly through your living space, creating a healthy and welcoming habitat promoting wellbeing and success.

Or perhaps you are more familiar with the **prana** from Yoga and the Indian system based on chakras connected through nadis (meridians) through which the prana flows nourishing the body with energy. Or the **ti** of the Hawaiians who believe the leaves of the ti plant have divine powers as it is filled with spiritual power.

Most cultures acknowledge the energy all around us and within us in some way. Even modern medicine reflects this network of highways through which electric signals and energy flows: our nervous system and the fascia (muscle sheaths) along which the neurons are transmitted communicating with the movement of the body and maintaining homeostasis.

Whatever you call these channels: **meridians, nadis, fascia**... they all transport the **energy / prana / ki /**, etc. and this entire process starts with the breath. The inhalation of air whether you believe that "prana rides on the back of the breath" or simply that we need oxygen to live, it is this visualisation of the source of energy entering our body and filling our centre of energy that forms the basis for understanding Reiki energy exercises.

You will be able to see some similarities between Reiki and Tai Chi or Qigong or Yoga because they all involve meditative practices and focusing on channelling energy to improve one's health and wellbeing.

Yes, Reiki is a spiritual system – please don't get stuck on this point. As explained below, it does not involve having long hair, singing "om" around a crystal grid and eating vegetarian sausages for dinner.

---

[1] (Source: Wikipedia)

From a scientific point of view we can quantify the energy that surrounds us in terms of vibrations. Everything vibrates, everything is therefore energy.

Energy - The Law of Vibration[2]

The Law of Vibration states that anything that exists in our universe, whether seen or unseen, when broken down and analysed in its purest and most basic form, consists of pure energy or light which resonates and exists as a vibratory frequency or pattern. All things, even thoughts and feelings have their own vibrational frequency. The thoughts and feelings we choose have their own specific rates of vibration. These vibrations resonate with other matter or processes that have an identical frequency. In other words, "like attracts like". If you think good thoughts, more good thoughts of a similar nature will follow and the same applies in reverse. The resonation goes further than this as you will also be in vibrational harmony with others who are like-minded. Most of us are familiar with the concept of the "Law of Attraction".

Science has shown that everything we know in the universe is ultimately made up of units of energy; these quantized units vibrate at specific frequencies. Quantum physicists have proven that although matter appears to be solid, when looked at through a high-powered microscope, it is broken down into the smallest possible elements: molecules, atoms, neutrons, electrons and quanta (the smallest particles measurable). This reveals that matter is mostly empty space interspersed with energy. We could therefore logically assert that everything is made up of energy and empty space. Everything that appears solid is in fact the result of the vibrating frequency of the energy that makes it up.

This is where the art of creative visualisation and manifesting your goals as visual thoughts begins. If you allow or train your *conscious* mind to

---

[2] (Source: weebly.com)

reflect on thoughts of a certain type as a matter of habit, over time these will become an integral part of the *subconscious* mind. The vibrational frequency of these types of quality of thought will become the dominant vibration of your mind-set. This is the resonance you will be working off of in your attitude and in the way others perceive you. You will be drawing in others with a similar quality of dominant resonance. This also applies vice-versa as you pick up on the "vibes" that others around you are emitting.

If they are within your field of energy (either physical or emotional) they can become intertwined with your resonance, with your energy. On a chemical level, people or couples who have been together for a long time tend to have higher levels of oxytocin (bond forming hormones usually present in pregnant and lactating women to strengthen the bond with their child) in their posterior pituitary gland. In much the same way, if you are around someone who is positive for a long time, you will feel their positivity rub off on you and someone with negative thoughts, negative resonations, will start to drain you and disturb you energy field. You create "bonds" or "chords" as they are sometimes known, that attach you.

Whatever you are feeling creates the template for your vibration. In essence, this is a definition of our conscious perception of vibration. Because you cannot see it does not mean it is not there.

Just like with a music fork. Tap music fork A and it will begin to vibrate and resonate. Those waves of energy/vibrations travel outwards. If music fork B is in the energy field emitted by Fork A it will start to resonate as well – try it!

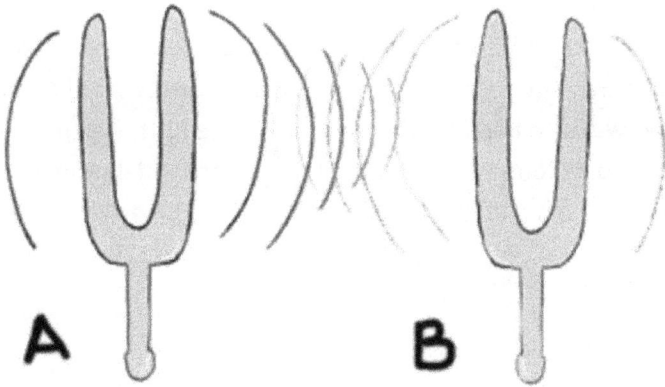

A   B

To become a great athlete and reach your maximum potential, you need to understand the infinite source of energy that is around you and within you. How this energy literally affects you and becomes intertwined with you. It can be the energy of others and/or the energy around you created by other matter. The art of channelling this energy is not some ancient tradition practiced by mystic hermits up in a mountain in some far off land, it is a gateway open to us all to allow us to restore balance in our minds and lives.

The modern world may be hectic, but it doesn't mean we have to be part of that rat race. We can be part of our own race. We have choices. I believe it is a wise choice to be open and to heal yourself, to make sure the life you live is the best life you could possible have. One that you are proud of. If you want to get fit, if you want to win that marathon or lose weight and be health for the rest of your life: heal thyself, learn how to use this energy!

The art of channelling energy in modern terms

Looking at an "alternative" therapy through the terms used in modern Western therapy helps to break down the hocus pocus boundaries and prejudices we have been conditioned with since birth. The modern face of Reiki could be loosely explained through more widely known and accepted concepts and therapies, such as:

- Creative visualisation

- Getting rid of brain junk

- Emotional release / anger management

- Positive thinking

- Meditation

The above concepts and therapies are based on the same elements that make up Reiki:

- Visualisation

- De-cluttering

- Channelling

- Intent

- Focus

To get started, I am going to ask you to expand your "frame of knowledge" – don't worry it is not painful, at least not in the physical sense! I am asking you to open your mind essentially to concepts you previously were unaware of or thought were not possible because they were not accepted by the general consensus of belief.

An example of this "frame of knowledge" would be the well-known misconception of people believing the earth was flat and that if we walked to the horizon, we would fall off the edge. Thanks to new experiences, findings and technology we shifted this frame of knowledge to a new one: the earth is round!

I am asking you to view Reiki in much the same way. It may be something that is not known to you or something you have categorised as hippy gobbledegook. Either way, if it is outside of your "frame of knowledge", please exit your comfort zone and open your mind to allow it to benefit you. Think in terms of meditation, channelling your negative emotions into something positive, creative visualisation and getting rid of brain junk.

As exemplified in the previous section: Everything is energy. Reiki deals with this energy, which most of us cannot see and yet we are surrounded by this energy. Everything is made up of tiny atoms that are vibrating. This vibration creates energy.

The first law of thermodynamics states:

> *"Energy can neither be created nor destroyed –*
> *it can only be altered."*

This is key to Reiki. Just as when a psychotherapist asks a patient to channel their anger or negative emotions into something positive and constructive, the therapy revolves around the concept of emotions having an energy. Our body holds onto this negative energy at a cellular level, what we call "bottling up our emotions". At some stage, we then "explode" if we do not give these negative emotions a way to be released back out of us, such as through physical exercise, shouting, singing, crying and so on.

We cannot see the energy held in these negative emotions but we feel the way they manifest as we become short-tempered or sad or bitter. Reiki teaches you how to move this energy (both negative and positive) in order to balance out your energy inside you. You draw the energy around you through visualisation and channel it into your body through visualisation. Result: a balanced energy system. A balanced disposition.

Your fixed "frame of knowledge" in this respect is screaming that is not possible. You are conditioned to believing that only weirdoes believe in the mumbo jumbo of invisible energy and yet millions of you are prepared to accept the concept of creative visualisation advocated by motivational gurus such as Tony Robbins. So let's keep an open mind.

Your new "frame of knowledge" should now be able to integrate the following:

Reiki balances your own energy system getting rid of negative energy such as fear, anxiety and worry through visualisation, focus and intent.

Now let's learn HOW to channel your energy to find out how Reiki can offer tremendous power in assisting you achieve your goals.

2 fundamental parts of energy channelling – already used by athletes, just phrased differently

We can start by taking your mind on baby steps through the whole process of energy channelling and base it on techniques already known and used by athletes:

1- THE BREATH

We've all seen athletes use breathing as part of their technique to power themselves around the racetrack or lift seemingly impossible weights above their heads. Yoga forms a bridge from these "accepted" techniques to the "alternative frame of knowledge". How many times have you heard Yoga instructors say: "Let the breath move you."?! Inhale as you extend, exhale as you contract. You may also be familiar with this technique if you go to Pilates, lift weights and all kinds of other fitness techniques.

This concept of the breath facilitating movement sounds a little more wacky if we coin the phrase used by Yogis: "The life force around us "prana" enters our body on the back of the breath". It is essentially the same "frame of knowledge" though. Moderating your breathing technique will improve movement and endurance. In brief, we have a "hocus pocus" way of phrasing the same concept that is scientifically and widely accepted: i.e. if you breathe erratically when you run, your body does not get enough oxygen in to supply the bloodstream and muscles, this will mean the body creates lactic acid sooner, making you burn out sooner. Simply put, you will also be out of breath sooner. The source of energy starts with the breath – whichever way you phrase it.

2 – FOCUS

A second familiar technique is that of <u>focus</u>. Let's expand that concept a little further to include other mental factors such as a desire to succeed, confidence and determination. All these mental factors are drivers to achieving your goals. They are drivers, which I will nicely bundle into the concept of "motivation". Without motivation you cannot control all the other "physical factors" such as training, eating habits, general lifestyle, relationships, mental preparation and sleep. The physical and mental factors work together.

We accept the need for a successful athlete to have "determination", which is ultimately a part of the whole concept of motivation. In Reiki, the determination is referred to as "intent", i.e. the desired outcome you want, the goal you are focussing on, the end game you want to achieve. That intent and determination are honed through the regular practice of Reiki. The easy 3-step daily energy exercises (12-15 minutes a day) will eradicate all other riffraff distracting your mind from your intent, and leave you with just your priorities.

Your "frame of knowledge" in terms of Reiki as a breathing and focussing technique can now start to incorporate and accept the concept of energy channelling. This is not a physical process. We use the art of visualisation as a means of focus, intent and determination. These three mental factors are all composites of motivation. To succeed in your training or rehabilitation, you need to be motivated. Others may be there to support you, ultimately though it is your own motivation that is the main driver in both mental and physical terms.

To recap:

Breath is the beginning. It is our source of power.

Focus and intent on priorities, our end goal, form our motivation.

How to practice Reiki

How does it work?

Find a quiet place where you can sit undisturbed for 15 minutes.

Focus on your centre of energy (this is traditionally the tanden in Japan, just below your navel, or it can be your solar plexus if you follow the chakra system – I am not going to force this issue) and you perform meditative techniques.

These both calm the mind and assist in bringing your body's energy system and thought process into balance, into harmony.

Simple daily exercises - that use your breath, but don't leave you out of breath:

- are designed to clear and cleanse your energy
- they ground you
- deepen your experience of and connection with energy
- bring your own energy system into balance
- build up your personal reserve of energy

Part 1. Preparation: Clearing the energy around you.

Part 2. Meditative sequence to help you focus on your centre of energy*

Your energy centre is the centre of your being, source of your power, creativity, intuition and much more. It is drawn upon in many well-known oriental practices such as martial arts and meditations.

It is said that your energy, your ki is moved by the mind: "... where the attention goes, ki flows..."

By effortlessly focussing your awareness on your centre of energy (your tanden) equates to you placing your energy there. The tanden is the base where you will be working from.

ENERGY REBALANCING EXERCISES

Here is the breakdown with diagrams to make it even easier for you.

First sit down comfortably – personally I feel it doesn't matter how you sit as long as your back is straight and you are comfortable.

i) – Preparation You may light a candle or incense if this helps to get you in the "mood", i.e. whatever acts as a trigger so you know it is time to quieten down for 12-15 minutes.

Start with your hands in your lap, palms down.

Focus on your centre of energy. Inhale and exhale deeply 3 times. (You may keep your eyes closed for this if you wish).

ii) – Cleansing Now you will begin the energy exercises starting with a purification ritual (origins: Tendai Buddhism).

'Dry Bathing' or 'Brushing Off' to get rid of negative energy.

Rest your right hand on your left shoulder/upper chest, and as you exhale run your hand down your torso to your right hip.

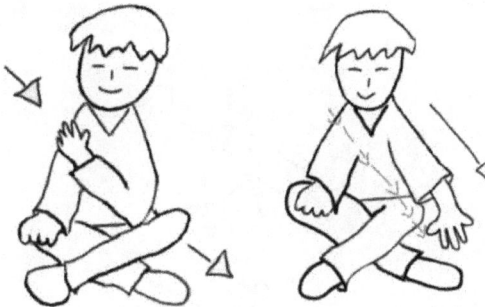

Now do this with your left hand (resting on your right shoulder), and finally repeat with the right hand again.

Next, brush along your arms.

Start with the right hand on the left shoulder.

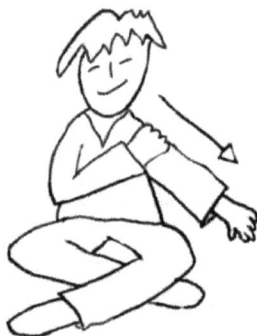

As you exhale, brush along the outside of your left arm and past your fingertips, exhaling as you do so.

Do this with your left hand on your right arm, and then finish by repeating with the right hand again.

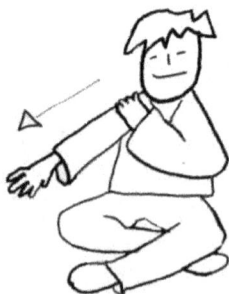

iii) Connect To connect to the "universal life force" that surrounds you, close your eyes and turn your palms upwards (you can raise your arms above your head or keep them at waist level, whatever suits you).

Visualise energy flowing into your hands (maybe as a beam of light or simply a sensation) travelling into your body through your palms into your centre of energy where it builds up. Do this for a minute or two until you feel the sensation or become aware of the connection on your palms and are happy with a firm visualisation or sensation of the energy travelling into you.

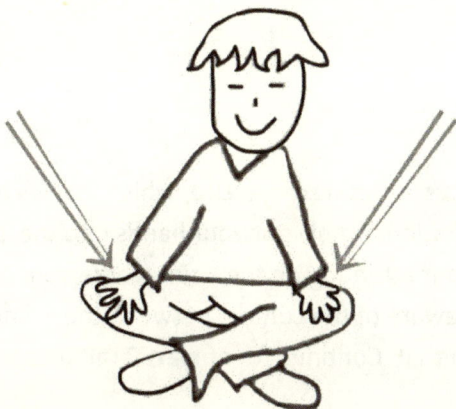

iv) Purification Breathing Method - to balance and boost your energy.

Place your hands on your lap with your palms facing upwards and breathe naturally through your nose. Focus on your centre of energy and relax.

When you breathe in, visualise the energy (this can be a beam of light) cascading into your crown and passing through your body to your centre of energy. As you pause for a microsecond before exhaling, feel that energy expand throughout your body, melting all your tensions. When you breathe out, imagine that the energy surging out of your body in all directions. Repeat for at least 3 minutes. You are now a conduit of energy. Like a bamboo cane.

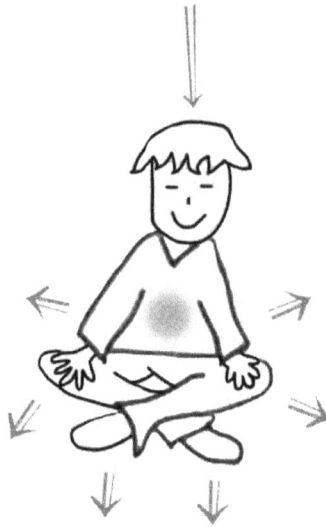

v) Meditative focus In this next exercise, which follows on from the purification meditation, simply put your hands into the 'prayer' position and gently rest your attention on the point where your middle fingers are touching. Be aware of the contact between these fingers and focus your attention on that. Continue for at least 3 minutes.

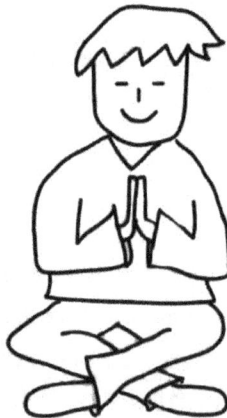

vi) Channelling energy Keeping your hands in the prayer position, you will now start "channelling" the energy. When you breathe in, pull energy through your hands and take the energy straight through your abdomen to your centre of energy.

Feel the energy increasing, building up and when you breathe out, push the energy from your centre of energy out of your hands again. Repeat for at least 3 minutes. Establish a smooth flow in and out or your hands – in and out of your centre of energy.

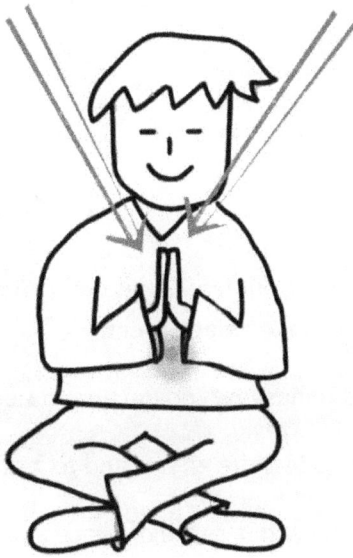

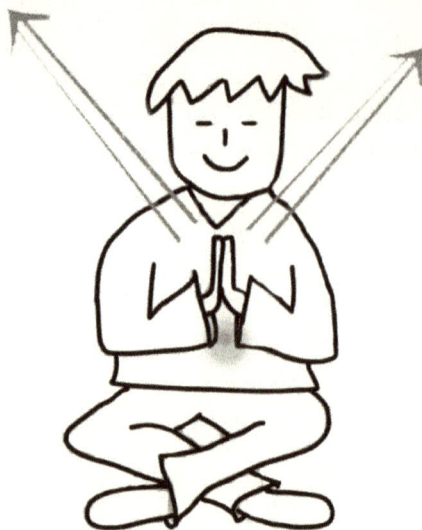

Finish

Place your hands back to your lap, palms down. Acknowledge internally that you have finished. Take a deep breath.

Open eyes and shake hands up & down/side to side to "disconnect".

Take a few moments to feel the effects and to feel grounded again.

Then go forth and shine with a sense of peace and balance and inner strength.

Part 3: Mindfulness As you can see these daily energy exercises use the energy around you to generate benefits for yourself through visualisations, meditation and focus. But there is another fundamental cornerstone to traditional Reiki, that of cultivating your own mindfulness. Mikao Usui offered 5 precepts to live by in a strive for balance and harmony).

Mindfulness can be assisted by adopting just a few precepts to learn to live by:

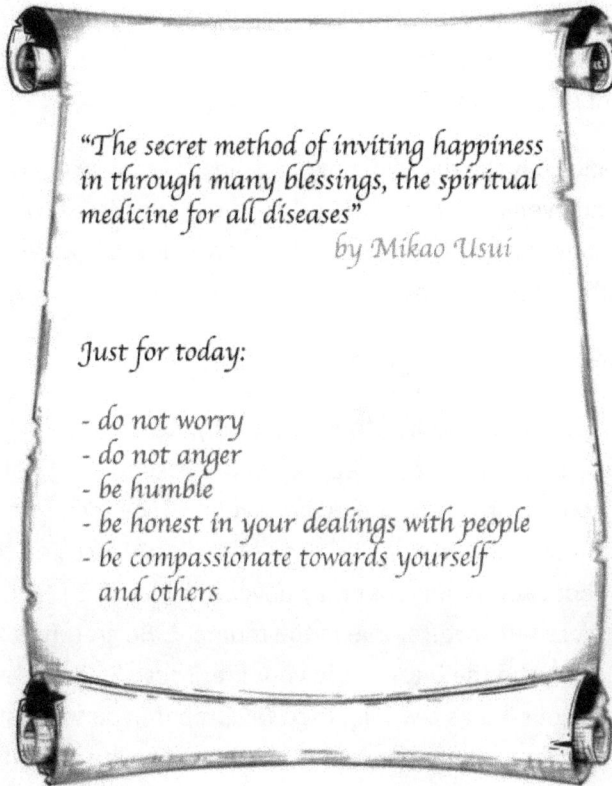

> "The secret method of inviting happiness in through many blessings, the spiritual medicine for all diseases"
> by Mikao Usui
>
> Just for today:
>
> - do not worry
> - do not anger
> - be humble
> - be honest in your dealings with people
> - be compassionate towards yourself and others

These guiding principles are not based on religion but it must be mentioned that they are founded on the Japanese doctrine of Shugendō dating back to the 7th century, which literally means "the path of training and testing" or "the way to spiritual power through discipline."

Now that you have the steps and the knowledge with which to start your journey to inner harmony and balance you must remember that in order to truly succeed at anything involves an element of discipline.

Regular routine (everyday)

Make Reiki part of your daily routine (there is an assisted video/audio on YouTube for the daily energy exercises: www.youtube.com/watch?v=LLS4e1KxgSY).

In this instance it is the discipline of practising Reiki once or twice a day (morning and evening) 12 to 15 minutes. These exercises flow through the breath, but don't make you out of breath –they are not what could be called difficult or exerting!

The rest falls magically into place.

Practice mindfulness (also no lifting required!). Keep things in perspective. Remember the 5 precepts, perhaps keep a copy at your desk or on your refrigerator, somewhere you will see them. Do not dwell on past, pointless distraction. Do not endlessly focus on the future and worry about something that may never happen. This is illusory and akin to needless self-torture. Live in the moment. Be grateful for what you have. Recognise the blessings in your life. These 5 precepts will not only improve your life as a whole, they will prepare you to master getting fit - the ideal figure and/or performance you are aspiring to.

If your mind wanders during your meditation, don't worry, just bring your thoughts back gently to settle on your centre of energy. Like in the film "Eat Pray Love", the calmness will come over time. The character played by Julia Roberts has a preconceived idea of meditation being an easy switch-off. It is not. It is more like sucking on a cough sweet and feeling it smoothly melt away in your mouth over time. Allow your erratic thoughts to be the cough sweet.

You will not achieve the perfect meditative state in the first week. Don't expect to "feel" anything either. You are sensitising yourself. It is a learning process. Example, if you could speak French you would not need to go for lessons. Everything comes in time.

Reiki is more than just meditation. Over the course of time, with regular practice, it will make you more aware and sensitised to the energy around. There are certain "sensations" you may already be able to feel, such as a "tingling' in your hands or cold/warm air over your palms.

How to feel and understand Reiki

Remember, just because you cannot see it does not mean it is not there.

You cannot see air and yet you need it to breath and stay alive. You cannot see the millions of bacteria living on the skin of your very own body and yet they are there!

Trust me (and thousands of others), this is not the Emperor's New Clothing!

Here is an exercise to give you a palpable sensation of the energy that surrounds you:

Rub your hands together vigorously for 20 to30 seconds, as though you have just come in from the cold. You are already feeling heat between your hands, this is energy. It is a transformation of kinetic energy (movement) into thermal energy (heat). To feel how far this energy reaches or how far it extends from your hands in an outward direction, place your hands about shoulder width apart and by pulsing your hands (palms facing) gently together and apart you will notice where the thermal energy field from one hand meets that of the other hands as you sense a kind of "bouncing" effect. For best results close your eyes to remove visual stimulus and try to sense the energy as a physical entity.

There is nothing preventing you from placing your palms together. The point of the test is to "feel" the energy that you cannot see, as we sometimes only believe in what we can see. Asking you to practice energy channelling exercises in order to improve your fitness and help you attain your ultimate goals is asking you to take a huge leap of faith if all this is new to you and you cannot even "see" what you are channelling.

Much like this "bouncing" effect you can feel between your palms, as if you were pulsating around something spongy and squishy, from the thermal energy you have created, you constantly have an energy field around you.

Some people call it an aura. These "auras" vary in depth reaching out from just millimetres from your body to whole metres. From the "etheric" layer, which is closest to our physical body – these we clear during dry-brushing at the beginning of our daily energy practice in order to remove imbalances before they manifest in our physical body.

Greater clarity. The next concentric layer is the "emotional" layer, which is self-explanatory, it is where your emotions resonate, followed by the "mental" layer, which is said to hold our ego, how we identify ourselves as distinct form other things and beings through our own ideas, beliefs and experiences. Finally, before the spiritual layers, the "astral" layer acts as a boundary between our practical everyday awareness and spiritual nature. This is where our fears, paranoia and sense of disorientation originate if the energies are not in balance here.

Our outermost energy fields are the spiritual bodies: "celestial" and "causal". It is here that we begin to draw in the universal life force, the energy that we merge with in order to harness it and reach our ultimate goals and potential – not in the sense of the "ego", but in the sense of everything working harmoniously together. All our energy field "bodies" transcend into pure energy when they merge with this natural universal energy surrounding us. Here we tap into the real magic, the raw power. Channelling this into your own centre of energy when you are in a balanced and clear state is the moment when you soar.

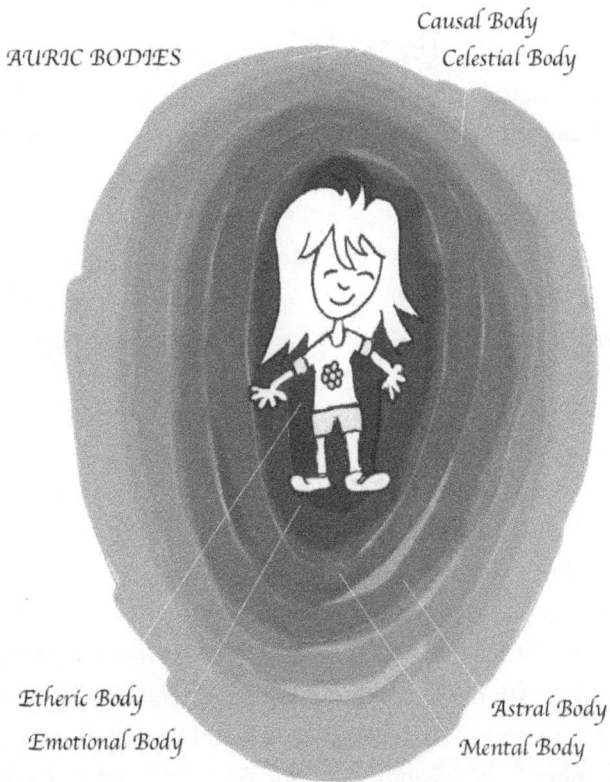

AURIC BODIES

Causal Body
Celestial Body

Etheric Body
Emotional Body

Astral Body
Mental Body

(Etheric –> Emotional –> Mental –> Astral –> Celestial –> Causal: these are the main energy fields we give off through our "vibrations" that are usually denominated as our "auras".)

It is important when decluttering your mind in preparation to focus and in order to achieve clarity of thought that you appreciate and acknowledge the fact you have auras/fields of energy around you.

In your daily exercises, the first of the 3 steps is to cleanse yourself of negative energies. This is known also as dry-brushing. You are moving your hand through the energy around you, removing static and unwanted energy before proceeding onto the first exercise of purification: channelling new energy through your body.

Below are the steps used by Reiki masters and practitioners to self-heal. It is extremely useful if you feel like you are carrying around a lot of emotional baggage in the form of regret, depression, self-loathing, emotional trauma, stress, suffer from insomnia, anxiety, depression... it is best to get yourself in balance, i.e. to heal yourself, before starting on the journey of attaining your maximum potential. We should always work from a strong foundation otherwise we will have nothing to stand on when we reach the top as our foundations crumble away.

Please note that depending on the extent of your "baggage" or trauma, you may need to seek additional assistance and you may also experience what is known as a healing crisis. For some this is only minor, perhaps feeling sleepier because their body needs more rest to rebalance, others may feel a huge shift in their eating habits, breakouts on their face, sleeping for 10-12 hours a night, trust me though it will pass if you are consistent with your self-healing regime (again just 15 minutes a day). When you come out the other end of your healing crisis, you will be "balanced". Your energy levels will be where they should be, you will be more focused and confident in your decisions and thoughts.

Self-healing

What to do – a step-by-step guide to self-treatment

During this meditation you will be effortlessly focusing energy onto five areas of your head – shown below. Try these different approaches to focus the energy. Find the one that works best for you. Eyes closed. Sitting comfortably.

(1) Duplicate self-treatment: Visualise yourself (a duplicate of you) sitting on the floor with your back towards you. In your mind's eye, see your-self treating your duplicate, with energy flooding out of your hands into the various areas of your duplicate's head or simply energy flowing in (no hands).

or

(2) Imagine your duplicate self is standing behind you, treating the "real" you.

Imagine energy or light flooding out of your duplicate's hands into different positions of your head.

or

(3) Simply visualise the energy flowing into the 5 positions (no hands) listed below.

or

(4) Imagine that you are being treated by disembodied hands, with energy or light flooding out of these hands into the 'real' you.

or

(5) Don't visualise anything at all, but allow your attention to rest or to dwell on the different areas of your head.

The energy will follow your focus and direct itself where your attention is directed.

Your intent and your focus are the essential factors in this simple method.

Below are the positions to visualise energy entering your system for self-healing

(1) Front of the forehead along the hairline.

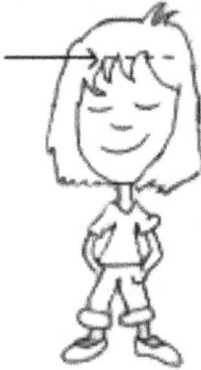

(2) The temples.

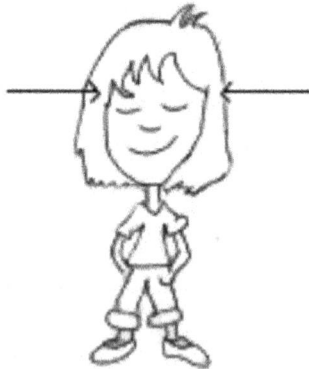

(3) Front of the forehead and the back of head.

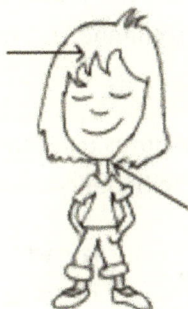

(4) Back of the neck and the base of the skull.

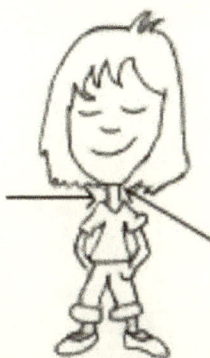

(5) The crown.

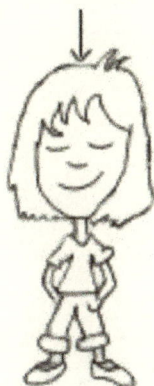

This method of self-treating is deceptively powerful, and can be carried out whenever you have even a few minutes to sit still with your eyes closed and imagine the energy channelling into your body's energy system.

Ideally you might spend 3-5 minutes on each position, but even 1 minute for each position will be beneficial.

The important thing is to self-treat **regularly**. Once you feel at ease with yourself, you can self-treat at longer intervals if you don't have time, you must however continue with your meditative daily energy exercises in order to keep your sensitivity to the energy around you and you're ability to tap into this energy and let it flow through you.

The Benefits of Reiki for an athlete

Balance and homeostasis

Homeostasis: it is something we do naturally. It is essential if you want to be healthy. Being healthy is essential for your training and fitness success.

Finding harmony is an inert characteristic of being human, we learn this in biology at school. The systems in the body are all designed to seek and establish balance, to work in unison to keep us alive.

Back to school: Elements and conditions within the body are controlled/auto-regulated, to provide a constant and stable internal environment. This is called homeostasis. The conditions and elements that need to be controlled to ensure this balanced state include: body temperature, water content, carbon dioxide level and blood sugar level.

Whether you call them the brachial plexus, lumbar plexus, solar plexus, lumbar plexus, etc. or chakras, we have energy centres and systems in our body that all work together, they are vital centres for your overall wellbeing. Reiki helps us re-establish this system of inner balance as well as transposing to the way we see the world and our own life.

Although different cultures have different ideas on where the centres of energy are, they all acknowledge we have a base "centre of energy".

In traditional Japanese disciplines dealing with spiritual, therapeutic, martial or artistic methodologies, there are 3 centres of energy (see diagram below). Reiki focuses on the lower tanden (Seika Tanden), which is scientific terms is your body's centre of gravity (The upper centre of energy is between the eyes and the middle centre is at heart level.)

Centres of energy
in traditional Japanese disciplines

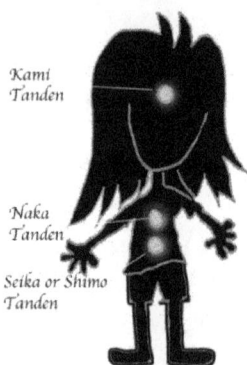

Kami
Tanden

Naka
Tanden

Seika or Shimo
Tanden

Centres of energy
in traditional Chinese disciplines

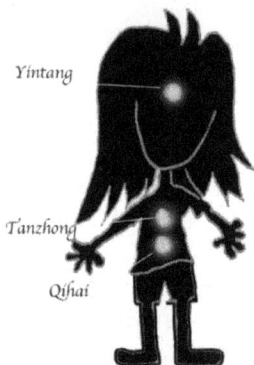

Yintang

Tanzhong

Qihai

Centres of energy
in traditional Indian disciplines

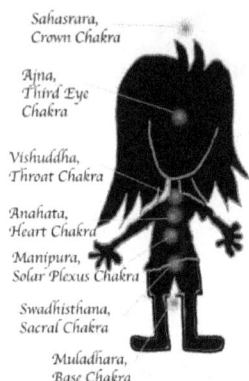

Sahasrara,
Crown Chakra

Ajna,
Third Eye
Chakra

Vishuddha,
Throat Chakra

Anahata,
Heart Chakra

Manipura,
Solar Plexus Chakra

Swadhisthana,
Sacral Chakra

Muladhara,
Base Chakra

As you can see from the second diagram, the Japanese system is based on the Chinese system. The latter is well-known in the field of martial arts where for centuries they have been using the lower dantian (the "ocean of qi") as an epicentre for explosive power, also referred to as the "second brain" for its intuitive and kinaesthetic role. Qigong, for example, has long focused on the lower dantian in particular because when it is properly looked after, it creates a strong, grounded and robust individual full of raw energy. As with the Japanese practice of Reiki, all centres of energy within the body must be healthy for a balanced mind and body to work in harmony giving an athlete that competitive edge.

In India, the "subtle body differs slightly, with centres of energy referred to as your "chakras" – receptors and distributors of life-energy. The diagram below illustrates the 7 main chakras and it is your solar plexus chakra (Manipura) that is considered to be the centre of dynamism, energy, will power – but this system too meditates on the Manipura to attain power.

In scientific terms a nerve plexus is a network of intersecting nerves; nerve plexuses are made up of afferent and efferent fibres that arise from the merging of the anterior rami of spinal nerves and blood vessels.

Amazing how people got things so right before dissections and x-rays came into use:

Plexus:

1. any complex network of nerves, blood vessels, or lymphatic vessels

2. an intricate network or arrangement

Word origin of 'plexus'. From Latin plectere to braid, plait

These nerve plexuses are specific hubs providing connections and information to other parts of the body. As in the "subtle body", they all work together to keep your body in balance, to maintain homeostasis.

Reiki channelling is one way of keeping all this energy flowing smoothly and maintaining the balance. What happens when the body is not balanced? There is the risk of disease, infection, and illness. Just take one of these conditions, e.g. temperature. If your body's temperature is not maintained/regulated within the relatively narrow limits of approx. 35°C to 41.7°C (95°F to 107°F) this can result in a heat stroke if the body gets too hot or hypothermia if it is too cold.

Stress

A big factor affecting the body's ability to maintain homeostasis, i.e. a balanced state inside the body is stress. The whole process of homeostasis relies on signals being sent to the various systems of the body telling them, in the instance of temperature for example, the hypothalamus sends signals to cool down or warm up. This all starts with sensors, so for example you might start shivering if the temperature drops (your body is contracting muscles to generate heat) or if you're too hot you sweat to cool your body down. If you are "stressed" and in a constant state of "fight or flight" with worrying thoughts making you pump adrenaline around your body, this will block essential signals being sent to certain systems that need looking after. For example, in a state of stress your nervous system is getting the body ready for danger, for an attack – even though there is no real mortal danger in front of you. This shuts down flows to systems that are not needed when you are about to "fight" something, e.g. your digestive system. If this system becomes "neglected" for too long it will not function properly as it will not be receiving the nutrients and signals it needs. These signalling airwaves (nadis, meridians, nervous system, etc.) need to be flowing and open to help the entire internal organisation of your body communicate and work efficiently and effectively.

If we see balance as the fortress of your internal body, stress is like the enemy from within that lets the drawbridge down weakening your defences, inviting in the enemy and illness.

Reiki as a motivator and performance enhancer

Repeating the daily exercises will naturally help you establish your priorities as superfluous actions

and habits fall by the wayside since they no longer serve you, meaning they have a negative impact on you so you release them.

Improve the quality of your life and relationships. Help temper your expectations and the way you interact as well as your emotions.

Reiki energy channelling can be used as a much more powerful form of motivation and performance enhancer.

By working regularly with Reiki, you can reap the benefits. It has the potential to make a huge difference in your life. Predominantly a calming effect. you will feel calmer, more positive, better able to cope, stressful situations and negative people will not affect you as much. You are less "reactionary". You can see situations and people with greater objectivity.

All of this is not an overnight transformation. You will notice positive changes as time goes by; when you look back over a few weeks, you will notice you are reacting differently to life and situations.

Key benefits of Reiki:

1. **Clarity**. Reiki helps you to cut through the rubbish and see your priorities with clarity:

Working out your real priorities. Reiki gives you impetus to arrange your life so you can focus on what is important to you. This may in turn make you feel upset or confused about certain choices you have already made. Have faith in yourself. You are feeding your "gut instinct". Your intuition resides in your base tanden/dantian/chakra. You are awakening it – your "second brain". That is why your reflexes will improve as well as you can intuitively pre-empt what is coming.

2. **Simplification**. Reiki will give you the strength to help you make the necessary changes. After this low you will be rising to your right path. Also simplifying your life on other levels.

3. **Healing**. Physical symptoms may need to be released. It affects sleeping patterns. My "healing crisis" lasted 2 months – with a lot of sleep!

It brings it to balance. Releases things you do not need: physical, thoughts etc. Each person's reaction is personal.

The energy is moving you in the right direction.

4. **De-stress**. Stress is at the root of a lot of illnesses. Reiki de-stresses.

Okay so it de-stresses me and gets me focussed, how is this going to help me get fit!?

Without being weighed down with the baggage of worry and stress and the superfluous, you dedicate more energy and focus to your fitness regime. By having a clear mind you realise (some or all of these may apply to you depending on your reasons for wanting to get fit):

- it is important to be healthy

- you do not want your life dictated by your injury

- you want to excel

- you want to be your best

 - you want to realise your full potential

- you get rid of the lethargy

Lethargy can be your biggest enemy in terms of motivation. This lack of enthusiasm and energy is reversed with Reiki. It rebalances your energy. So in physical terms you have more energy you no loner have troughs of fatigue. It naturally brings with a desire to change your diet (a whole other discussion!) so you tend to desire the right foods, no longer want to binge eat, probably eat less or no meat, a balanced body and a balanced mind means there is no longer a rejection or blockage to exercising.

Channel energy and focus with Reiki in your training. Fuel your intuition. Become more sensitised to the energy around you.

Although the whole concept of Reiki revolves around "spiritual" development and "self-healing", the technique and precepts of Reiki energy channelling can used as an art for focusing your mind on what you want to achieve.

While some of you may still believe all this spiritual healing is nothing but hocus-pocus, it would be foolish to ignore this simple technique. It is a simple technique anyone can benefit from to improve his or her life. It can help you to focus on almost any goal you want – for the purposes of this guide we are looking at how it can help you achieve your fitness or rehabilitation goals – through visualisation and intent. As you now know, the latter two techniques are easy to learn.

In hindsight you will "see" the effects of Reiki.

Remember, you may not notice anything at all happening as you practice Reiki, however, I guarantee that when you look back over a few weeks or months of regular practice, you will see a huge difference. Fewer bad habits, focusing on what is important to you, improved sleeping patterns, greater clarity and focus, more confidence, increased intuitive perception and a happier, more relaxed disposition.

Now that you have a better understanding of what is involved in Reiki and its benefits, we can move on to music as a motivational factor and performance enhancer.

2 - Music

The power of music

Unlike with Reiki, we do not need to expand on music's general history, as we are all aware of what music is. I will though ask you to give a thought to music in its various guises not just as some great sounds to jig around to at a nightclub or in your bedroom!

The different guises of music include:

- a form of expression

- to create an atmosphere and feeling

- an integral part of celebrations and festivities

- a medium for relaxation and soothing

- a powerful healer

Music in its various forms has an irrefutable effect on our behaviour. It can make us want to get up and dance, reduces us to tears, makes us feel elated or comforted, assists us in communicating – the list is almost endless.

It is the music, even more than the spoken word that holds this power to move us. It transcends all languages, it brings back memories of smells, tastes and feelings, is used in psychotherapy, as a birth aid, to help cope with grief, war chants to create fear, sonorous exercises to heal our organs through vibration, in meditation to calm the mind and promote wellbeing – music is a law unto itself.

To help us on our journey to fitness, let's take a look at that the relationship between music and physical performance, and what exactly music does when we use it as part of our training.

(For the sake of ease I am going to call you the "athlete" in some of the explanations below – if you don't feel like one now, you will by the time you finish this guide!)

MOTIVATION

Music has been used for motivational purposes and therapy for many years. Just as it is the result of a great creative power, whether this creativity stems from love, passion, hate or envy - it is also is the source of great power. As Armstrong so eloquently put it in his poem on "The Art of Preserving Health, 1774":

"There is a charm: a power that sways the breast

Bids every passion, revel or be still,

Inspires with rage or all your cares dissolves,

Can sooth distraction and almost despair –

That power is music

Music exalts each joy, allays each grief,

Expels disease, softens every pain,

Subdues rage or poison or plague."

We can already see the overlaps here with Reiki. Music as a mood changer, music as a healer and music as a source of energy.

Music influences a person's mind, body, spirit and emotions. This means that music can almost control our state of mind. In this respect there is little doubt that music affects our **motivational levels** to varying degrees depending on a person's personality and the type of music being played.

Motivation is a key factor in exercise. It can push us or guide us towards an end target or goal as an external outside stimulus, just as you can motivate young children to do almost anything for you with incentives such as sweets or prizes! Some people do not need the aid of external stimulus as they are motivated by the love and passion of what they want to achieve. I am sure even they may need a helping hand somewhere along the line.

Music is not always "motivating" though. It is able to work its way into our minds and hearts to stir emotions like no other medium, but by the same token, for the purposes of exercising, listening to music without motivational qualities (such as depressing lyrics or a funereal melody) can have an adverse effect on our training. Sad music or songs with negative lyrics will still be effective as an external stimulus and motivators, but they will not act as **positive motivation**.

The definition of "positive motivation" in the context of this guide is based on "psychological processes that cause arousal, direction and persistence of voluntary action that are goal focused"[3] - sound familiar with regards to Reiki? This is our "intent" and "focus". It is as though music awakens the kundalini in us - the dormant serpent of energy that lays coiled at the base of our spine according to Hinduism. Music arouses this dormant serpent and as it rises and uncoils we become energised, we move away from a state of despondency and lethargy. The effect of this can be seen quite clearly at rock concerts or the opera. The music stirs the audience to tap their feet, clap their hands or cry and laugh. It awakens our energy. This effect on your mood before and during exercise therefore has an impact on your motivation levels. The psychological effects music has on our mood states can be just what we need to shift from a sad to a happy state, making us more likely to train after listening to music or knowing that we will be listening to music as we train. If the playlist we listen to during exercise is uplifting we associate this state of happiness with our exercise session. Just like

---

[3] Mitchel 1982, Gardener & Shah (2008), p 235.

when you might crave chocolate because it releases those happy hormones (endorphins) and you associate it therefore with feeling good, in the same way you will associate your training sessions with this "feel-good factor" and naturally want to repeat them.

When it comes to exercise, music has behavioural and psychological effects on both men and women that are constant and measurable. When chosen appropriately with the desired effects in mind, music has a positive impact on performance by increasing endurance and psychological states such as motivation and greater effort. The music selected should also be suited to the athlete's socio-cultural background and age group so they can "relate" to the music. For example, there is no point playing rap to a female in her 50s (demographic studies show men prefer rap or hip hop, heavy metal and electronic music, whereas women affiliate more with pop and pop rock - source: musicstats.org) as it will either have no impact on her motivational levels or the reverse impact: de-motivation.

Be warned, research shows that working out to music you don't like can actually make exercising feel harder!

Your playlist should match your type of workout! (See page 53 for some suggested playlists)

When selecting music to motivate an athlete, we not only need to make sure we choose gender and socio-cultural-specific music, we must also consider the exercises to be performed and the desired heart rate. According to studies, a tempo of 125-140 beats per minute is the ideal range for aerobic-based, cardio exercise for most healthy participants.

Add the factor of motivational and relevant lyrics and you're well on your way to breaking through barriers and setting new records – or simply surprising yourself - for example 'Fight Song' by Rachel Platten, 'The only way is up' by Jazz and 'Keep on running' by the Spencer Davis group.

Motivation is a variable factor that affects performance in sport whether it is an individual or team sport. To be the best you can, you need to keep your motivation at a constant. Peaks and troughs in motivation both during away from exercise will not bring out the best results. If you feel disheartened or despondent, you will not go to the gym or push yourself to your limit. It is important to be motivated to get the best out of your performance. That is why is important to integrate music into your fitness/exercise regime as a "complementary" therapy and driver. Remember, Reiki and music approaches fitness from a holistic approach. Fuel your soul as much as your muscles for ultimate results.

Don't forget, you must make sure that you choose the right kind of music. Motivational music (as described above) affects your levels of motivation when you exercise, to the extent of eliciting greater ergogenic effects during endurance-based exercises than with simply "neutral" music or music that may not be appropriate in terms of socio-cultural and age factors.

Without listing the numerous case studies researched over the years, it is clear that music can well be used for motivational purposes, that the tempo and genre of the music play a role as well in motivational terms. Being more "motivated" helps athletes change their attitude and mind set. They will want to be healthier and eat healthy foods. They will want to focus on attaining their end goal. This notwithstanding, does music actually **enhance performance directly**?

There is plenty of research to support the claim that the effect of music on exercise actually works: Chipman, (1966) proved that music increased the muscular endurance of college students completing a sit-up test; a further study[4] of women in a press-up test evidences the same. There is also proof from Beckett (1990) showing that college students were able to walk faster and further with less effort whilst listening to music than without. These facts back up music as a direct motivational factor in helping athletes improve their performance –

---

[4] Koschak (1975)

listening to inspirational music while you train has a positive effect on your results. Being more motivated will help you reach your goals quicker and want to maintain them, rather than being unmotivated, without drive and seeing exercise as a chore rather than a pleasure.

Music as a motivator makes you "want" to
exercise as opposed to "need" to exercise.

Further proof that music undeniably gives you a competitive edge can be substantiated through the ban of headphones and ipods at the 2007 New York marathon for fear that some athletes (those listening to music) could have an unfair advantage over others – there was some mention of the ban being enforced for health and safety reasons too!? This ban caused an uproar among the runners who mostly trained and ran with headphones! Because of the psychological effect that music can have on individuals, depriving them of the music can have a detrimental effect on their performance, like putting lead weights in the shoes of runners who are used to running whilst listening to music.

We have seen how music can motivate and work as an external stimulant in exercise, now let's look at its ability to put you in a state of dissociation, i.e. it distracts you from the exertion thereby permitting longer and more intense training than without this "distraction" or state of "disassociation".

DISASSOCIATION

Disassociation is a psychological effect that stops us feeling and thinking that we are exhausted. Music is definitely distracting as any of you who have tried reading while listening to a song you know can testify: cognitive learning is impaired when listening to music. If you are studying and listening to your favourite music you are less likely remember what you read than if you studied in silence. Again it must be stressed that listening to music directly, i.e. through headphones has a stronger impact than just listening to "background" music, which acts less as a distractor. If you listened to music before studying and relaxed, i.e. countered the effects of stress, this will increase your ability to retain the content of your tasks.

Researchers have found that that an athlete's rate of perceived exertion can change as a direct result of the music they are listening to[5].

Furthermore, wearing headphones blocks out the sound of us breathing and our heart rate, this in turn will stop us feeling tired because the sound of our breath and the speed of our heart rate can psychologically slow us down. Headphones block out the signals sent to the brain telling it the body is tired and needs to rest.

This state of disassociation leads to what is known as a lower Perceived Rate of Exertion – i.e. we don't notice we are tired as much. Latest statistics show that the average Rate of Perceived Exertion is lowered by as much as 15% when athletes listen to music whilst training or performing – usually in moderate intensity cardio or endurance exercises.

Dissociation occurs when an individual concentrates on external stimuli (the music) thus reducing the awareness of internal bodily cues such as heart rate and breathing rate therefore a reduction in the rated of perceived exertion that regulates how tired you feel. An interesting

---

[5] Haulk and Turchian (2009)

change is the oxygen uptake in relation to synchronous music: due to the nature of the music influencing the rhythmicity of the movement, a lower oxygen uptake is apparent due to the physiology of the movement – meaning your cardiovascular system does not have to work so hard and other systems in your body are less strained as a consequence. This is the same effect as meditation. It is said that our consumption of oxygen can decrease up to 20% when we meditate!

There are further physiological effects of rhythmic exercise on a non-elite athlete: listening to music whilst exercising not only helps us exercise for longer (improved endurance), it can result in ergogenic gains, improve performance and have a considerable positive effect on our anaerobic performance. Great news!

In summation, **BEFORE** training, music in its guise of "creating an atmosphere and feeling", "a medium for relaxation and soothing" and as "a powerful healer" de-stresses you to prepare you to perform at your best instead of being in an impaired state when you approach your training. Music also distracts you and motivates you **DURING** training and enhances your performance and gains because you are more likely to push yourself further in this motivated state. Music fuels the desire to want to train because it is enjoyable.

PREFERENCE & TEMPO

We have touched on the fact above that music genre is also a factor that affects motivation and therefore, in holistic terms, determination, focus, intent and ultimately performance. The genre of the music can have an impact on your levels of motivation as can your music preference. You may be listening to the right rhythmic music at the right tempo for the exercise you are doing but if you don't actually like the music you are listening to.... you aren't exactly going to be motivated (or perhaps, you are motivated to finish quicker!)

Accredited researchers[6] have alluded to findings demonstrating that music preference is also significant in the effects it has on exercise. They even go one step further to include the preferential differences between males and females stating that males prefer more bass compared to the more lively music preferred by females. They also found that situational context has a massive influence on the effects rendered by music, e.g. athletes have preconceived ideas on what music should be played on different occasions and in different environments for the respective training sessions. In brief, the type of training or exercise dictates the type of music athletes want to listen to.

Listening to your favourite music can encourage you to perform better due to the effect that liking the music has to your arousal levels. Research also shows that music promotes a positive attitude towards exercise, as does preference[7]. The studies included interviews with college students who had enrolled in an aerobics class: 97% of the these students said that music helped to improve their performance in class.

Music preference can affect the results of your performance, as you are more "positively motivated" to music you like compared to music you

---

[6] Hargreaves and North (2008)
[7] Fella (1988), based on 70 college students

dislike. Returning to the holistic approach of whole body and mind, it has been shown that listening to your preferred choice of music reduces anxiety levels[8]. Reduced stress enables athletes to perform better because they are i) healthier, ii) more focused and have increased drive. Based on tests on randomly assigned subjects in aerobic dance with two groups[9] - one listened to their preferred choice of music and the other did not listen to any music - the results showed that group listening to the music they liked achieved the best results.

But it's not that simple. We need to take a closer look at the tempo of the music. We already know that tempo has an impact on the type of exercise and training. There is also research out there showing that listening to our favourite music does not necessarily culminate in improved performance. The relationship between music preference, exercise and heart rate is a nonlinear one, showing inconsistent results due to a number of inflections[10].

On the one hand there is research confirming upbeat music motivates and has better results, and on the other there is research showing that the genre of music had different outcomes. So you need to make sure your choice of music suits the exercises you are doing.

There is evidence showing that when it comes to walking or jogging on a treadmill, athletes fatigued later with more soothing and soft music compared to fast louder music[11]. This could have been due to the beat of the music and the effect that it has on heart rate. Not all music motivates us in the right way.

A further investigation on the effects of fast and slow music on a 500m sprint in rowing found that fast tempo music showed the best results in terms of the time it took to complete the sprint[12]. It also found that the

---

[8] Mok and Wong (2003)
[9] Dwyer (1995)
[10] Karageorghis et al (2007)
[11] Copeland and Franks, (1991)
[12] Rendi, Szabo and Szabo (2008)

number of strokes per minute increased with the music (both fast and slow) compared to the controlled group with no music. In conclusion to this test they claimed that music acted as a psyching-up stimulus in short and strenuous muscle work, with a faster beat giving best results for this kind of training.

So where does that leave us... do not fear! It's all in the rhythm. In order to achieve the best results, the tempo of the music you listen to must be matched to the type of exercise you are performing – plus it needs to be music you like and synchronous, as proven by the study below:

Karageorghis & Simpson (2005) conducted a 400-metre sprint study (as cited above) where non-elite sports persons (males with an average age of 20) were tested on the treadmill performing a 400-metre sprint with i) synchronous music, ii) neither motivating nor de-motivating music and iii) no music. The results showed that the synchronous music had the best results. Synchronous music provides a beat that the athlete will unconsciously synchronise with when performing therefore if it's an up tempo best the athlete will keep to the pace[13]. Furthermore synchronous music will benefit repetitive exercise like treadmill running and rowing due to the nature of the exercise and the extent that exercise can last for.

Now let's make some specifically designed playlists and get motivated!

---

[13] Kerageorghis et al (2011)

Here are some playlist examples supporting this factor of tempo

Cardio / Strength Training
Tempo: 120-145 BPM

"Animals" by Martin Garrix	128 BPM
"Sail" by awolnation	120 BPM
"Seven Nation Army" by The White Stripes	125 BPM
"Wild" by Jessie J featuring Big Sean	129 BPM
"This Is What It Feels Like" by Armin van Buuren	130 BPM
"Sweat" by Major Lazer ft Laidback Luke & Ms Dynamite	130 BPM
"Clarity" by Zed featuring Foxes	128 BPM
"Crackin" by Bassjackers	128 BPM
"I Need Your Love" by Ellie Goulding, Calvin Harris	128 BPM
"Blurred Lines" by Robin Thicke ft TI & Pharell	120 BPM
"Levels" by Avicii	126 BPM
"Hey Now" by Martin Solveig + The Cataracs ft. Kyle	128 BPM
"Pour It Up" (Cosmic Dawn Remix) by Rihanna	130 BPM
"Right Now" by Rihanna, Julian Jordan, & Martin Garrix	128 BPM
"I Need a Hero" by Bonnie Tyler -	**148** BPM
"We Found Love" by Rihanna	128 BPM
"Marry the Night" by Lady Gaga	128 BPM
"Hall of Fame" by The Script ft. will.i.am	**136** BPM
"Tsunami" by DVBBS & Borgeous	140 BPM
"Take over control" by afrojack	130 BPM
Danza Kuduro" by Don Omar	130 BPM
"You Make Me Feel..." by Cobra Starship ft. Sabi	132 BPM
"Helena" by My Chemical Romance	126 BPM
"Dance Again" by Jennifer Lopez featuring Pitbull	128 BPM
"Good Feeling" by Flo Rida	128 BPM
"Up and Up" by Haddaway	132 BPM
"Give Me Everything Tonight" by Pitbull	129 BPM
"Scream and Shout" by will.i.am ft. Britney Spears	130 BPM

Cool-down / Warm-up / Yoga
Tempo: 60-90 BPM

"Over the love" by Florence and the Machine	70 BPM
"Spaceboy" by Smashing Pumpkins)	60 BPM
"All of me" by John Legend	82 BPM
"Possibly Maybe" by Bjork (Lucy Mix)	60 BPM
"Teardrop' by Massive Attack	89 BPM
"Dog Days Are Over" by Florence and the Machine	75 BPM
"Written In The Stars" by Tinie Tempah ft. Eric Turner	**92** BPM
"Lovesong" by Adele	60 BPM
"Me & Mr. Jones" by Amy Winehouse	89 BPM
"Missing" by Beck	90 BPM
"Salt Skin" by Ellie Goulding	90 BPM
"I'd Like To..." by Corinne Bailey Rae	90 BPM
"Nice Dream" by Radiohead	60 BPM
"Burn" by Ellie Goulding	**88** BPM
"In the Waiting Line" by Zero 7	80 BPM
"Down" by Marian Hill	85 BPM
"Come away with me" by Norah Jones	80 BPM
"Sweet Jane" by Cowboy Junkies	84 BPM
"This Woman's Work" by Kate Bush	66 BPM
"You don't own me" by Grace ft. G-Eazy	63 BPM
"Heathens" Twenty One Pilots	90 BPM

Now when you make a playlist not only will you be super keen to try it out, you know you're going to get the results you want from your training! It is positive all the way.

NB Remember to keep changing your playlists around and adding new songs to keep you inspired. For more songs, including running playlists, visit **www.heavenlyki.com.**

Music as a motivator and performance enhancer

Music can motivate. Disassociate and distract. Help us forget we are tired. Lower our rate of perceived exertion. Make us look forward to exercising, transforming training and weight loss from a chore into a fun activity we look forward to. And now we know it directly influences our performance.

LES MILLS workouts

The inspirational LES MILLS workouts are the perfect embodiment of music as a motivator and performance enhancer for all the reasons explored above. These include the GRIT- HIIT cycle workouts, BODYATTACK or the more gentle sessions of BODYFLOW and BODYBALANCE. Their system is based on choreographing moves and poses to suitable music in order to maximise the intensity and effectiveness of your workout.

Carefully selected inspiring and amazing tracks with the right tempo and lyrics to suit the respective exercise have been successfully designed to "Reduce Stress. Match Your Goals". The Les Mills family has pioneered this creative and innovative winning formula over four decades, and it is stronger than ever with their proven workouts as a firm fixture in clubs throughout the UK, e.g. the David Lloyd clubs found in 86 towns across the UK. They championed workouts "driven by the beat of modern music" – loved by all generations. In addition to these world-renowned fitness workouts there are numerous studies to support the claim that music directly improves your performance during exercise. This includes a personal favourite of mine: Zumba!

Here is a study (courtesy of the Sport Journal) illustrating just this point without dwelling on all the variables such as backgrounds, music chosen etc.:

STUDY: THE EFFECT OF MUSIC LISTENING ON RUNNING PERFORMANCE

"The purpose of the study was to investigate how listening to music while running affects performance Twenty-eight undergraduate kinesiology students at Texas A&M University-Corpus Christi (17 males, 11 females; age = 22.9 ± 5.9 yrs) were studied to determine if running performance was affected by listening to music. Running performance (RP) was measured by a 1.5-mile run. Two trials were performed, the first was a running performance without music listening (RPWOML = 12.94 ± 3.35 min) and the second trial was a running performance while music listening (RPWML = 12.50 ± 2.48 min). [...] Statistical analyses determined a significant difference ($p < .05$) between running performance without music listening (RPWOML = 12.94 ± 3.35 min) and running performance with music listening (RPWML = 12.50 ± 2.48 min). [...] the results of this study indicate that music listening has a significant effect on running performance during a maximal 1.5-mile run. [...] Based on the results of this study it is recommended that coaches, athletes, and traditional exercisers consider listening to music during training to enhance performance."

Working off the premise of these findings and previous research, we can safely confirm that music can be used for motivational purposes - just how this should be prescribed must bear various factors in mind. Remember that the music should be fitting with the socio-cultural background and age of the listener, along with the desired effects of the music in relation to the type of exercise being performed. For example, if the exercise that is to be performed has a nature that is fast and the athlete needs to be highly aroused, then the music should pose the qualities to help him or her achieve this (higher tempo and motivational lyrics, in a genre of their preference, listened through headphones).

<u>Final thoughts:</u>

In essence we could affirm that

1 - we should listen to our "preferred" music in order to keep us motivated, when we are not exercising. Music off the track and out of the gym is also important in helping you reach your goals as it has positive effects on your training and relaxation, which will impact on your exercise performance.

2 - listen to the "right kind" of music whilst training (tempo in keeping with the training: warm up, yoga or full-on cardio, etc.). The latter helps us to break through boundaries. Make sure the lyrics aren't depressing!

Each time we break through what we thought was our best, we reach another level. This is how we build up our fitness, improve our performance. Through disassociation, i.e. a distraction as offered by music (with headphones in particular), we won't even notice we are getting fitter! The beat and tempo of the music can have physiological effects due to the beats of the music; it reduces anxiety levels; fast music raises our heart rate and blood pressure, whereas slow music has the opposite effect[14]. We need some types of music to soothe and motivate and other types of music to stimulate and disassociate.

Now let's see what happens when you pour the power of music and Reiki into the melting pot and take a daily dosage.

---

[14] Armon (2006)

3 - Symbiosis of Reiki and Music

Empowerment to reach your full potential

This is where the magic begins.

Thanks to the healing powers of Reiki, you are calmer. Your mind is decluttered, you've gone through the mental clearing out phase. You can focus on the job at hand. You want it to happen. You want to succeed. You are being true to yourself. No more junk food, no more feeling sorry for yourself. No more "I can't" moments.

On top of this you are balanced within. Your energy flows evenly. Those bouts of fatigue are a thing of the past. You are sleeping well. You are at ease with yourself and the world you live in.

If you have been doing your daily energy channelling exercises you will be able to draw on the power all around you. Not only are your energy levels already up, you can increase them as and when you need to throughout your regime.

The studies carried out for this book and by others have shown irrefutably that athletes who have integrated music as a motivational tool in their training regime have achieved better results than those who trained without music. If we then couple theses results with the power Reiki has given you, the whole world is open to you. The realms of infinity are yours for the taking.

Reiki focuses your mind on your end goal and music propels you there effortlessly, like a bird in flight.

Flying. That is the feeling you will get when you reach your peak performance. Like a cheetah engaged in its chase, your feet no longer touch the ground. Your entire body is working in unison, each and every cell working in harmony to the same beat of the music towards the same end goal. Your body becomes alive. You are a conduit of energy. Channelling it from the outside through your breath, fuelling your centre of energy. You blast through your comfort zone. You transcend the barriers of your physical self and those imposed by your fearful ego or your protective ego. When you reach your pinnacle you are selfless. You merge with the energy around you and soar.

How to apply Reiki and music during exercise:

As motivators, music will already get you to the gym and Reiki will have kept you centred – clear mind, healthy eating habits, balanced approach to life. Now what happens once you get to the gym or your place of exercise….

"Intent" and breath.

You will no doubt have seen top athletes focusing intently on their end goal, whether it is a finishing line, high jump bar or just to keep steaming past all the other runners in a long-distance race. Coupled with controlled breathing so that they can not only focus their mind but also fuel their muscles, they are working at an optimum level. With Reiki fitness you will take this process further.

As explained in the first chapter, each visualised breath will bring in the natural life force energy around you and fuel your own centre of energy. As you run or push or lift or whatever exercises you are fighting through, you will be able to visualise the energy streaming through your body and channel it down the fascia around your muscles. In "hippy" language we are talking about taking in the qi, the prana and feeding it down your meridians and nadis giving you natural extra power. You will feel the power surge through your body when coupled with the "disassociation" effect created by the music. You will not be performing at an optimum level, you will transcend that level like that streamlined cheetah.

Let music take you to the highest level, steady at that new higher momentum or weight without even realising it, you begin your "visualisation", moving the energy in and out of your body.

When you hit your "edge", channel the energy from around you to help give you those "wings", power your own energy system with the energy around you. By visualizing the energy coming in from around you your mind resonates with these "images", you feel alleviated, you feel the extra power. Keep channelling the energy, maybe as a light travelling down your spine into your centre of energy with every inhalation (just as in your daily energy exercises) and propel this bright light of energy through every limb and cell of your body as you exhale. Repeat. Continue this cycle until you have reached your target or completed your exercise.

Imagine you are a battery connected to the energy all around you charging off of its power. This power enters your body through the breath. The focus on your inhalations and exhalations will also focus the mind. Fewer distractions mean every action and communication in your body is maximized on the end goal – on that finish line, on pushing past your edge or on holding your position for just a little longer.

Every time you go beyond what you think is your "edge" your limit, your maximum and sustain it for 5, 10 or 15 minutes. this then becomes your next level of "normal". You start at a higher level the next time you train. This is what we would call improvement! Just like the body builders tearing their muscles each time (don't worry, it is microscopic damage) to then build on that muscle next time after it has repaired and grown.

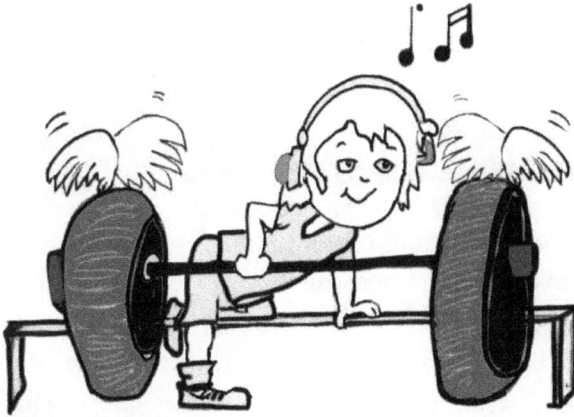

Give your workout wings

Training will become your joy not your chore.

Because you feel so great after your training, you will hunger for this feeling. It is a self-feeding cycle. Going beyond what you think you are capable of gives you such a natural high, a feeling of euphoria with the release of endorphin and dopamine hormones. Endorphins interact with the receptors in your brain reducing your perception of pain and triggering a positive feeling. Dopamine is a "pleasure" chemical, which makes us want to repeat whatever induced its release – a second helping of exercise please!!

The sense of balance from Reiki keeps you calm and focused on your priorities. You will want to exercise and not try to forgo training.

The music will also keep you motivated. Favourite songs off the track or out of the gym will keep your spirits uplifted even before you start training!

Despite differing and limited study results out there regarding music as a direct factor or performance enhancement and a distraction from actual energy exerted, I believe most of us would hand on heart say that we look forward to our jog or workout because we are listening some groovy tunes on our headphones. Right?

Basic level achieved through Reiki and music

Even if you are a sceptic on scientific grounds, there is irrefutable proof that people exercise more because they can listen to their music while they do it. Reiki prepares your mind-set in much the same way. Because you are more balanced and less stressed you actually want to do your training or exercises – with the added bonus of being in a healthier state to do this.

In this light, we could say that music and Reiki are motivators when it comes to exercise, rehabilitation and getting fit. Motivation is important in life as without motivation there is no desire to achieve. To be successful in your training motivation is crucial. In some cases you may need to be extremely dedicated and put in a lot of hard work to achieve the results you want – so you will need to be motivated! Daily energy, meditative and channelling exercises provide you with a calm level-headed mind frame from which you can approach your training without feeling it as a hopeless challenge, rather as something you *want* to do. By decluttering your brain and helping you be true to yourself, you are better able to focus on what is important in your life without it being a struggle.

Higher level

On a more intense level Reiki and music can also be seen as an ergogenic aid, another example would be caffeine or sports drinks – lets keep it legal!). Ergogenic aids (i.e. something that gives you a mental or physical edge while training or performing) are used in sport to help athletes be successful and music can be one of these. Music has been used to motivate for many years and now it is apparent that the use of specific types of music can have desired effects psychologically.

The use of music with headphones can provide the illusion of being in your own little world and the loudness of the music means that disassociation will be apparent. Research from Karageorghis and Terry (1997) has shown a result of this can lead to a 10% decrease on rate of perceived exertion thus giving us a psychological edge. And because you are better able to draw on the energy around you and your own personal energy system is more balanced, you can use the visualization of Reiki to channel more energy through your body when you most need it, when you are at the "edge" or need to boost yourself around that final lap.

Using simple breathing techniques, coupled with the visualisation of drawing energy into your own centre of energy, you can channel energy into your body from that infinite source of universal life force that is all around you. Through this visualisation and your intent – whether it is to get up an impossible hill or lift an impossible weight – you merge with the energy around you and achieve your goal.

Final thoughts

Music is now used all over the world in lots of sporting situations to motivate athletes in pre competition, in competition and also during exercise. Furthermore, the types of music that are used can depend on the sport and also the personality of the athlete. There is evidence to show that music has psychological and physiological effects and this can be used as an advantage[15]. Research has shown the positive effects and advantages that using music in sport and exercise[16]. The fact that music was banned in the 2007 New York marathon shows that it can be used as an advantage against other competitors who do not use music.

No doubt music will continue to be widely used across all sports as a motivator for ergogenic gains. I sincerely hope Reiki will be added to this trend, to help athletes find holistic balance and improved wellbeing, as well as improve their fitness and increase their peak results.

Everyone at some point in life will feel the effects that music has on your thoughts, emotions and on some occasions, even your actions. Whether it be making you get up and dance, made your drive home bearable or finishing the house work quickly and efficiently, having the power to understand why this happens can help change someone's mood and actions in an instance. Hence the use of music in psychotherapy and rehabilitation. In sport the effects are just the same and prescribing music for training purposes has been proven to work and can be used as an ergogenic aid for years to come. There is evidence to show that music works and can be used as a motivation tool to improve performance[17].

Although Reiki may not have been originally designed to help us win a marathon or improve our physical performance, I am sure its founder Mikao Usui would not disapprove of its use as both as a motivator for

---

[15] Fisher, Goldfarb, Milton (2006) and Armon (2006)
[16] from Mok and Wong (2003) and Parker (2009), backed by Leslie (1967)
[17] Karageorghis et al (2007) and Dwyer (1995)

fitness and rehabilitation and as ergogenic aid to create high-performance athletes and help people on their way to recovery or weight loss. After all, they all have the same goal: wellbeing. Designed as a system for self-healing, Mikao Usui's system gives us the calm and level-headed attitude we need to find inner peace. it also gives us a platform from which we can go on to excel. By learning the simple daily energy exercises and living by the precept of not worrying, not getting angry, being humble, honest and compassionate you will keep life's main goals in sight. You will no longer be distracted by petty problems. Reiki keeps you focused on the bigger things in life and helps you towards them whether they are academic-based, wealth-focused or, for our purposes here, athletic.

Relying solely on yourself and your physical training programme to get you through rehab, or reach you desired weight loss or attain the fitness levels you want is not wrong, in my opinion though it is less fun and effective than embracing the benefits of music and Reiki.

So remember: All you need to do is 12 to 15 minutes a day of the energy exercises. I would recommend the self-healing treatments (or visit a reputable Reiki practitioner) until you come through the other side of your "healing crisis" and then just add these to your daily routine as and when you feel the need – when you feel out of balance, or as the usual saying goes, when you feel "out of sorts". Add music to your day, both in and out of the gym or on and off the track. Keep yourself happy, keep yourself motivated. Design your own playlist to suit your training and exercises (remember to keep it slow for the warm ups and cool downs). When you need an extra "boost" draw on the energy around you through visualization and intent. You will feel yourself flying as you merge with the universal life fore around you and its energy pumps through your body.

Reiki will help you focus your mind, to see your goals clearly, better align you with your true self and music will elate you and move you along this journey filed with the passion, power and inspiration of music.

Whatever your fitness goals may be, "Reiki and Music" will make the journey there effortless, fulfilling and rewarding.

Resources

Armon, Fisher, Goldfarb & Milton (2006). Effects of music tempos on blood pressure, heart rate, and skin conductance after physical exertion. Accessed on 23/3/2013.

Bacon, C. Myers, T. & Karageorghis, I (2008). Effect of movement-music synchrony and tempo on exercise oxygen consumption.

Beckett, A (1990). The effects of music on exercise as determined by physiological recovery heart rates and distance. Journal of Music Therapy (27) 126-136.

Bell, J (2010). Doing your research project. A guide for first time researchers in education, health and social science. Open University press, Berkshire.

Bjork, A (1975). Short-term storage. The ordered output of a central processor. Cognitive theory. 1 151-171.

Chipman, L (1966). The effects of selected music on endurance. Master's thesis, Springfield College. Completed Research in Health, Physical Education, and Recreation. (9) 462.

Cohen, C. Manion, L & Morrison, K (2007). Research methods in education. Routledge, Oxon.

Copeland, L. & Franks, D (1991). Effects of types and intensities of background music on treadmill endurance. The Journal of Sports Medicine and Physical Fitness 31 100-103.

Dawidowicz, P (2010). Literature reviews made easy. A quick guide to success. Information age publication inc. United States.

Dwyer, M (1995). Effect of perceived choice of music on exercise intrinsic motivation. America psychological association. 19(2) 18-26.

Edworthya, J & Waringa, H (2006). The effects of music tempo and loudness level on treadmill exercise. Effects of Music on Exercise Performance. 49(15) 1597-1610.

Feller, K (2008). Music components and styles preferred by young adults for aerobic fitness activities. Journal of music therapy. (1) 28-43.

Gardener, W & Shahn, J (2008). Handbook of motivation science. Guilford publications, Ink. New York.

Gorard, S (2004). Combining methods in educational and social research. Open University press, Berkshire.

Haluk, K. & Turchain, C (2009). The effects of music on athletic performance. Ovidius University annals. Series physical education and sports science, movement & health. 1(9) 44-47.

Karageorghis, I & Deeth, P (2002). Effects of motivational and oudeterous asynchronous Karageorghis, I & Deeth, P (2002). Effects of motivational and oudeterous asynchronous music on perceptions of flow. Journal of Sports Sciences. (20) 66– 67.

Karageorghis, I & Simpson, S (2007). The effects of synchronous music on 400- m sprint performance. Journal of sports science. 24(10) 1095-1102.

Karageorghis, I (1999). Music in sport and exercise: Theory and practice. The Sport Journal. 2(2). 214-220.

Karageorghis, I Jones, L & Low, D (2013). Relationship between exercise heart rate and music tempo preference. Research quarterly for exercise and sport. 77(2) 240-250.

Karageorghis, I Terri, P Bishop, A & Priest, D (2011). The BASES on the use of music in exercise. The British association of sport and exercise sciences.

Karageorghis,I Mouzourides, A Priest, D Sasso, A Morrish, J & Walley, L (2007). Psychophysical and ergogenic effects of synchronous music during treadmill walking. Journal of Sport & Exercise Psychology. (31) 18-36.

Karras, B. (1997). You bring out the music in me. Haworth press, London.

Koschak, P (1975). The influence of music on physical performance of women. Master's thesis. Central Michigan University. Completed Research in Health, Physical Education, and Recreation 19(99).

Leslie, J (1967). The effect of music on the development of speed in running. Master's thesis. University of Washington. From Completed Research in Health, Physical Education, and Recreation (10) No. 697.

Lidor, R Layyan, N Morrow, K Tonnel, S Gershgoren, A Meis, J. Johnson, M (2004). The effects of music type on running persistence and coping with effort sensations. Physiology of sport and exercise. 5(2) 89-109.

Mok, E & Wong, K (2003). Effects of Music on Patient Anxiety. AORN journal. (77) 396-397.

Mouzourides, P Sasso, M Walley, C (2009). Psychophysical and ergogenic effects of synchronous music during treadmill walking. Journal of Sport & Exercise Psychology. (31)18-36.

Cover page music graphics from
<ahref="https://pngtree.com/">pngtree.com</a>

Pelletier, I Fortier, M Vallerand, R Tuson, Briere, N and Blais, M (1995) Toward a New Measure of Intrinsic Motivation, Extrinsic Motivation, and Amotivation in Sports. The Sport Motivation Scale (SMS) Journal of sports and exercise psychology. 7(1) 35-53.

Rendi, M szabo, A & szabo, T (2008). Performance enhancement with music in rowing sprint. Sports psychologist. 22(2) 175-182.

Restle, M Shiffrin, J Castellan, R Lindeman & Pisoni, D (1989.), Cognitive theory. Hillsdale, NJ: Lawrence Erlbaum Associates. 1 151-171.

Ridley, D (2008). The literature review. A step by step guide for students. Sage, London.

Swim Science (2014). Reliability rating of perceived exertion in swimming.

Wilson, E (1883). Observations of an Italian exile. Mills, Jowett & Mills, London.

Wolf, L & Smith, J (2009). The Consequence of Consequence. Motivation, Anxiety and Test Performance. Applied Measurement in Education. 3(8) 227- 242.

My Reiki lineage:

Mikao Usui
Chujiro Hayashi
Hawayo Takata
Phyllis LeiFurumoto
Florence O'Neal
Jerry Farley
June Woods
Simon Treselyan
Marcus Hayward
Diane Whittle
Taggart King
Francesca Hepton

Acknowledgements

Firstly, of course, I would like to thank Jade for having agreed to submit her well-researched work on music as a motivator and its effects on RPE and dissociation to a complete stranger. She is testimony to the reason we all have faith and hope in humanity.

I would also like to thank my son Edward for having been my soundboard for all those unanswerable questions he addresses with logical simplicity and the understanding of a sage – not bad for a 16-year-old!

And of course my fantastic sister-in-law Melissa for having cast her scrutinising and objective eye over my work - I'd be lost without her - and my dear brother for his words of encouragement and belief... the fuel of all writers!

www.ingramcontent.com/pod-product-compliance
Lightning Source LLC
Chambersburg PA
CBHW031133020426
42333CB00012B/356